THE
FIGHTING
WINDS
of DESTINY

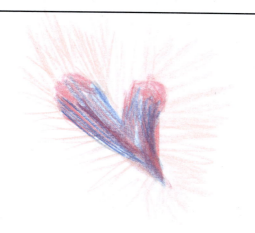

THE FIGHTING WINDS *of* DESTINY

The Amazing Story About Tough Times and Inspirations

Based on a True Story

ANITA NINA TESO

TATE PUBLISHING
AND ENTERPRISES, LLC

The Fighting Winds of Destiny: The Amazing Story About Tough Times and Inspirations
Copyright © 2014 by Anita Nina Teso. All rights reserved.

This book is designed to provide accurate and authoritative information with regard to the subject matter covered. This information is given with the understanding that neither the author nor Tate Publishing, LLC is engaged in rendering legal, professional advice. Since the details of your situation are fact dependent, you should additionally seek the services of a competent professional.

The opinions expressed by the author are not necessarily those of Tate Publishing, LLC.

Published by Tate Publishing & Enterprises, LLC
127 E. Trade Center Terrace | Mustang, Oklahoma 73064 USA
1.888.361.9473 | www.tatepublishing.com

Tate Publishing is committed to excellence in the publishing industry. The company reflects the philosophy established by the founders, based on Psalm 68:11,
"The Lord gave the word and great was the company of those who published it."

Published in the United States of America

ISBN: 978-1-63306-621-2
1. Biography & Autobiography / General
2. Biography & Autobiography / People with Disabilities
14.11.20

Thank you to those nice and wonderful people who surround me and make my life more meaningful. Thank you in advance to all my supporters who make my book possible.

Special thanks to these great people: Mr. Somnuck Teso, Mrs. Chalem Teso, Mrs. Lynne Raphael, Mrs. Cecelia Kirihara, Dr. Michael Somermeyer, Souvanna Kouanchao, Bong Xamonthiene, Sabaythong Vongkhaophet, Khonsavanh Kay Insisiengmay, Lyne Teso, Dr. Ketmani Kouanchao, Bryan Thao Worra, Laura Feld, and the nurses who have taken care of me.

INTRODUCTION

This story is about a person named Anita Nina Teso. Anita lived with three different families after she escaped from Laos to Thailand. She left Laos when she was very young. She and her family were the victims of war. Laos was once a French colony.

Life had been so tough on her that she had to work diligently for some people. But she had stayed a positive, quiet, strong, and respectful person. She was lucky to have the greatest brother of all, Xay, who had always been so supportive. She loved and highly respected him. He was a wonderful brother. Unfortunately, he passed away a few years ago, but he will forever be in her heart.

Anita loved to take accounting classes. She joined a two-year accounting program at Edison High School and graduated second place with 102 percent (tests plus extra credit for two years), from the program—not to mention the highest score for a minority student in business in 1987. She was very proud of the outcome.

She met and married a good man in 1992. Shortly after that, she conceived a healthy baby boy in 1993.

As a young girl, she has fought hard to survive. As an adult, she still has had to fight to stay alive. She found out that her kidneys were going to fail while she was pregnant with her child. After giving birth, she went for dialysis treatment three days a week for three hours each time. She did this after her shift at work. After being on dialysis for two and a half years, she got a kidney transplant on December 1, 2000. But her transplant kidney did not last long due to a reaction to the medication. It only lasted for a little bit over four years; she then had to go back to the dialysis unit for a second time in 2004. Hopefully, she'd be lucky enough to get a second kidney transplant in 2014.

Anita changed and reformed herself from a quiet, timid girl with low self-esteem into a strong woman with healthy self-esteem and self-confidence. Most importantly, she was a fighter. She had forgiven those who abused her emotionally, and she had moved on with her life with no regrets. She became interested in Catholicism and took a RCIA class. After finishing this class, she was baptized on Easter vigil at St. Gabriel the Archangel Catholic Church in 2011. She believes in God and in the virtue of faith even though her life is full of tests on intensity and endurance.

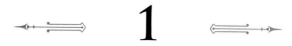

1

My name is Anita Nina Teso. I am an American naturalized citizen who was born in Savannakhet, Laos. All of my grandfathers and grandmothers were Thai citizens. My maiden name is Teso. *Teso* is for Thai. My paternity is both Laotian and Thai because my grandfather and my grandmother moved their family from Thailand to Laos. They took about one hundred people along with them to Laos, and they made their fortune there.

Many years later, my grandfather became ill and passed away. He left my grandmother in charge of everything. I saw my grandmother a couple times when I was young, but unfortunately, I never met my grandfather because he had died when my dad was young.

My father left his immediate family because he had sympathy for his mother, who had been working hard to raise and educate all of her children. He stayed with a priest and was raised in a Catholic church convent back in the old days.

When my dad became a man, he met my mother in Mukdaharn, Thailand. They married and lived in Thailand for many years. After they had several children, they decided to move to Laos. They had a total of fourteen children—five boys and nine girls. I am the ninth child.

My father joined the army and served for many years before he retired. After that he worked at the prison as a Wader and got promoted to a high rank of a warden. He worked in many prisons for some time before the new Communist government took over Laos and the French left the country.

My father's workplace was next to my school. I went there a few times with my friends, and I saw many strange things and many strange people while I was there. I knew from that day on it was not suitable for me or my friends to go over there anymore. My father was not rich; he was just a working middle-class person, but he was rich at heart. He helped a lot of prisoners become good people and offered help to those people who were in need.

One day, I saw several unknown people come to our house to meet my dad in person. I welcomed them by saying hi with a big smile, and then I walked away. When they left, I asked him, "Who are they and why were they here?" He told me they were his ex-prisoners and they had come to thank him and to express how much they appreciated everything he had done for them.

My father had a strong character; he was a tough man and was a prominent person in my city. I didn't spend a lot of time with him because he often traveled around the country, but I remember vividly the last time we spent time together. We went to see a movie. That night before leaving, he lit lots of candles around the house. This had something to do with a Buddhist holiday. He let me do it too. As a child, I remember all the wonderful times we had together even though it was just for an unfortunately short time. The lighting of the candles was also the last time that I had gotten attention from my dad. It was an unforgettable moment of my life. I was very proud of him, and he was my hero.

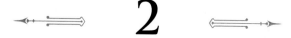

2

When I was three or four years old, my cousin came to visit my family. There was a big flood, and the bank in our neighborhood overflowed. She wanted to go to the next door neighbor by walking on the big wood plank that attached the neighbor's house to ours.

"Come on, follow me!" she called out repeatedly.

"Okay!" I finally said.

So I followed her, and I accidentally fell into that big flood. The water was up sky high, and I almost drowned. Luckily, I was saved by my favorite sister, who had me grab on to a tire tube. If not for her, I would not have survived that day.

Many years ago, I mentioned the incident about the flood to my cousin, but she did not remember that it was me who almost drowned that day.

"No, it was your older sister—not you," she said.

I replied, "Yes, I was that little girl. I have my sister as a witness."

She couldn't believe that I still remembered from the old days; she thought I was way too young to remember; even my sister had said so.

One summer day, when I was about four or five years old, I was alone when suddenly I saw a familiar face approaching me.

"Do you want to go with me?" she asked.

"No, I don't want to go with you," I replied.

Despite my protests, she grabbed me, and we got into a *sumlaw* (carriage). She told him to take off quickly before someone spotted her.

"Be quiet, okay?" she told me. "I'm going to take you for a ride."

I immediately obeyed. She was a family friend, and I didn't realize that she was kidnapping me. We took a bus for a few hours, and then we rode on a pickup truck for another few hours. She treated me nicely on the way to her hometown.

When we arrived at her house, her mother asked, "Whose daughter is this, and why did you bring her here?"

She told her mother who I was and that she really liked me.

"You cannot keep her here," her mother said. Her mother knew and highly respected my parents.

After that, she showed me off to her friends and neighbors. I was surrounded by them, and they told me how cute I was. They all seemed to like me because I was a cute city girl too.

The friend was very generous to me, but I didn't like her foods, drinks, and bed. Her mother seemed to notice my reactions.

It was on a Saturday night when she took me to the Buddhist temple by the river. She bought foods, candies, and drinks for me. It was some kind of annual celebration, so the temple was crowded with people.

When we returned from the temple, her mother looked at her and said, "You better take her home before she gets sick and before her parents come here to look for her."

I was afraid that she would keep me there forever; I missed my parents.

"Okay, I'll take her home tomorrow," she said.

Early Sunday morning, we left her house and she took me home. When she dropped me off, I remember exactly how my mother reacted. "Why did you take her without asking for my permission? We have all been looking for her."

"I came here, and she was alone. If I'd asked, you would have said no to me anyway."

"This time I will forgive you, but don't you dare do it again!" my mother exclaimed.

That was a last time I saw Keo.

My older sister, the neighbor kids, and I went swimming in the Mekong River one summer day when I was between six and seven years old. I almost drowned that day too. My sister saved my life by pulling me by my hair and dragging my body up from the bottom of the river. My mistake was having tried to go out deeper, not knowing how to swim. I was trying to follow the bigger kids who knew how to swim. My sister is only two years older than I am. I deeply appreciated her for saving my life that day. We kept this a secret from my parents because they never let us go swimming at the Mekong River without adult supervision. This incident was the second time I almost drowned as a young girl.

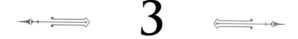

3

Unfortunately, toward the end of 1975, my favorite older sister, my younger brother, and I were sent to Thailand. A few days later, my brother and I cried like babies because we didn't want to stay in Thailand any longer. We were sent back to Laos eventually. As a matter of fact, I came to Thailand many times with my mom for a wedding and to visit my grandparents. I really enjoyed spending time with her. Until almost the end of 1976, one of my older sisters, Tiny, needed to escape from Laos, and she needed someone to hold on to her son while they were escaping. She had one boy, one girl, and a boy on the way. At the time, the oldest boy was almost two years old. According to Laotian laws, anyone under eighteen years old could go with their parents as a Thai citizen. On the other hand, if they were eighteen or older, they had to escape from Laos on their own, which was my sister's case. Apparently, I was not so lucky because she picked me to escape with her and her family.

I thought we were going to have noodle soup at my older brother's house that night. He was living by the Mekong River. When we arrived at his house, I was surprised because there was no noodle soup for anyone. Instead, I was forced into a small boat by my brother, and I couldn't do anything about it except yell, "No, I don't want to go!"

"Be quiet!" he demanded. "The soldiers are nearby, and they will shoot all of you at any time if they see you escaping."

I stopped yelling and became silent right away. While we were crossing the Mekong River, I was very scared because I couldn't see anything except the darkness. My older sister had grown up in Bangkok, so she knew how to speak Thai and she knew a lot about the country. I was young, timid, quiet, honest, and I was a respectful person at the time.

That was when a new journey of my life began. I was innocent and too young to leave home without my parents. I was so sad, terrified, and devastated. I cried quietly on the way there. Everybody was very quiet until an unexpected thing happened to us when we reached the middle of the Mekong River. Suddenly the water started to fill up the boat.

"Quickly, help me get rid of the water before we sink," my sister ordered, her voice filled with terror.

"Okay" I responded. I was holding on to my nephew and helping her at the same time. Surprisingly, we were able to manage it. When we came close to the shore of Thailand, we saw a fisherman.

"Where are you going? Are you coming from the other side of the Mekong River?" he asked. Everybody was quiet except my sister, who seemed to be in charge of talking.

"Yes, and we are going to our uncle's house," she responded.

"You'd better get out from the boat right now before the Coast Guard finds you and your boat sinks. How have you all survived in a small boat like that?" he said. He looked at us and spoke again. "I will take you guys to see the mayor. His house is not far from here."

After we all got out of the boat, my sister told him that we had many relatives living in the city because our mother was from the city too.

When we arrived at the mayor's house, the fisherman told him about us, and the mayor sent someone to get our uncle to pick us up.

I heard several people tell the mayor, "Their mother came here and told us to watch for her children because some of them had to escape from Laos due to their ages."

The Coast Guard appeared at the house and told the mayor that they saw someone escaping from Laos and they had spotted us from far away.

"Are these them?" the coast guard asked.

"Yes, they are" the mayor said. The mayor told him that we were Thai and our uncle was on his way to pick us up.

"If you say so, then we will not take them with us," they said to the mayor.

Just then my uncle showed up, and they left the house. Our uncle had a conversation with the mayor for a few minutes, and then he took us to his house. This incident has had a marked effect on my life, and I've never forgotten this life experience. This always comes to my mind when anyone asks me how I escaped from Laos. In fact, I didn't have to escape because I could have come with my mother and family freely without danger.

We were very lucky that a fisherman was very kind and gentlemanly to us. There were many horrible stories about Thai fishermen. It was well known that they sometimes promised to help people cross the Mekong River. After they have received payment and once they reached the Thai border, they would rob their passengers, flip over their boats, or kill the people and take their goods. There were so many unfortunate old people, young children, and pregnant women who died due to these attacks, their bodies left to float in the Mekong River. We could see bodies floating near the shore of Thailand almost every day. I felt very sad to see that, and I hoped none of them would be someone from my family or someone I was related to. In reality, there are good and bad people of all races in this big world that we are sharing. It does not only happen to Thai people, and it's absolutely part of human nature.

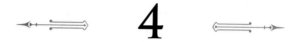

4

A little girl like me missed her parents badly. I cried every night for a long time, but nobody noticed it. I stayed with my sister and her family. At least I was so lucky that this brother-in-law was a very nice and generous person. He always took good care of me while I was staying with him.

One day, one of my brothers and his family came to town and asked me to live with them in Bangkok.

Why not just go live with them and do nothing? I thought. I decided to go with him, but I didn't know that I was making a huge mistake. I thought it would be a good opportunity for me to live with a new family and a chance to see a big city like Bangkok. It was the third time in my life that I had seen him because he was living with my grandparents in Thailand before I was born. I came from a big family, so I had a lot of brothers and sisters, but we did not grow up together because we were the victims of the war.

Bangkok was a big and beautiful city, but my life was not as pretty as I had pictured it out. It was a couple of days after we reached the city that I automatically became a babysitter. My job duties were to babysit three children eight to nine hours a day, Mondays through Fridays; to cook rice; and to walk about three miles to buy charcoal every week or two. Oh, I thought I just came to stay with them! I didn't expect things to turn out like this. Besides, I had never done anything like that in my entire life, especially that I had to cook rice the old-fashioned way for the whole family.

I had never cooked rice before, nor had I ever taken care of children. A hopeless person like me had no luck with cooking. One day, while I was draining hot water from a big pot, suddenly all of the rice and hot water fell on my left foot. I was in pain and was devastated. I cried like hell and worried about the disappointment I might receive from my brother and sister-in-law. I had mixed emotions while waiting for them to come home from work.

"What's a life?" I cried and said to myself. "I used to just go to school, come home and eat, study, and play with my friends. My parents would never expect me do these things!"

My brother later told me to smear toothpaste on my foot when I told him what happened. It was very painful. I suffered for many months. After that incident, my left foot became bloody, and it was soon replaced with new skin. Amazingly, I had no scar. I thank God for that toothpaste.

Despite all the troubles I've experienced, I had the courage to be a strong person and to be a positive person. At least I had one wonderful brother, Xay, who was always kind and generous to me. He gave me a little money to save every time he received his paycheck, and I saved all the money in a piggy bank. I felt very happy and thankful for his generosity. For a fourteen- or fifteen-year-old person, he worked so hard for his money. Sometimes I watched him working from a distance with tears in my eyes. He has passed away now, but he is always in my heart as the best brother that I ever had. He was a brother who always gave and never expected anything in return. "May God take him to a place where he belongs, such as heaven," I always pray for him.

One day, I received good news that everybody was going back to Mukdaharn for vacation. I was very delighted and so excited that I would have a chance to leave this family by going back to live with my sister, the one with whom I arrived in Thailand. Mukdaharn was very close to Laos, where my parents and family still lived.

An unexpected thing happened to me again. Before we left Bangkok, I discovered that my piggy bank had disappeared; someone had stolen it from me. I've never figured out how much money I'd saved. I said to myself, in tears, *There goes my first and only piggy bank. What kind of person steals money from a little girl?* I was speechless and unable to complain to anyone. All I wanted to do was to save up money for myself because of my living condition and situation.

Before we headed to Mukdaharn, we stopped at Ubon refugee camp to visit my oldest sister, Diamond. I was so delighted to see my sister whom I had not seen for a long time. She bought a blue and purple dress with a floral design for me. I didn't tell my sister anything about what had happened to me while I was living with my brother and his family. I was a very quiet and respectful person, and I didn't want to disrespect or embarrass them, either.

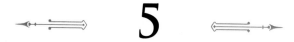

5

We stayed with Tiny in Mukdaharn about two weeks. Then my brother said that we had to return to Bangkok the next day. I got up early that morning. I didn't want to live with them anymore, so I planned to run away from them. Unfortunately, I met my sister-in-law on the way, and she tried to talk to me and dragged me into a carriage, but I refused to go back with her.

It made her very furious and disappointed. "I will tell your brother! You have to go back with us to babysit your nieces and nephew no matter what!" she said.

I ran away from her with my cousin because I didn't want to be found by my oldest brother. Later I decided to go to my uncle's house. I stayed with him and never returned to my sister Tiny's house. A few months later, I went back to look for my sister Tiny, and I discovered that she and her family had left the city. They went to Ubon refugee camp so they could come to the United States. They left without me, and they probably assumed I was okay staying with my uncle. I was fortunate that my uncle was a kind and generous person. His wife and most of their children were okay to me.

Once again, my life was not getting any better. I understood I had to help my aunt with the chores to show my gratitude. Some days I had to go to the market place to help my aunt sell vegetables with my cousin on weekends. I had to wake up very early in the morning to help sell jasmines to those who woke up early to give the morning alms to the Buddhist monks. I gave all the money to my aunt. Most people liked to tell me that I was too honest. I kept asking myself, "Why has everything happened to me this way, especially when my parents were not around to protect me, and what's a life, and why me?" I cried and talked to myself all the time.

Many times when I wandered and looked across the Mengkong River, I would cry seeing the roof of my home back in Laos, where my parents and my family were living. I was just a little kid, and I had no one else to rely on other than myself. Besides my uncle, there was one person who was very nice to me. She was my uncle's daughter-in-law. She paid me every time when I finished doing errands for her, and that was how I earned my money weekly. I appreciated her generosity.

One day, my other sister came to visit my uncle and stayed at his house for a few days. "Hello," she said.

"Hi," I said.

I was so happy to see my second older sister, Kay, because she left home when I was just a little girl. I had been very disappointed in the way I had been treated by Kay, who had not seen me for years.

After that incident, I was determined to work hard, study hard, and to be the best person I could be. I said to myself, *One day, I'll be successful.* I was attending school and started at second grade, and my then name was Nuntana Teso. I had proved to my uncle how much I loved to study by getting good grades. I knew he was very proud of me. It was the first time I attended school in Thailand; no one realized that I came from Laos because I could speak the Thai language clearly.

Life was precious and so unfair to me once again. During the school year, while I was riding a motorcycle on the way home from school, I accidentally fell off in the middle of the street on the way home. All I remember was my behind hit the ground. I was so afraid of getting hit by the cars behind me because it was rush hour at that time. The reason it had happened that way was because my uncle and I had stopped at the city's library and he had picked up too many books. I was the one holding them; they were too heavy, and I was too small to handle all the books. Nothing happened to me, and thank God for that miracle.

My cousin and I were about the same age. We became friends, but we were so opposite from each other. She was a leader, and I always was her follower. She took advantage of me and treated me unfairly sometimes while I was living with her family, but I couldn't say anything because she told me to be quiet. One day, a couple months before I reunited with my family, an unforgettable thing happened to me at my uncle's house. My aunt, my cousin, and her friend were having a small gathering without inviting me to join them. I was doing my chores in the kitchen.

It was about an hour later when my aunt came to me and asked, "Did you take my money?"

"No, how could I? I didn't go anywhere," I replied.

"My money was missing after I left those two alone with my purse," she said.

Here I was living with people who almost accused me of stealing money. There were three of them together. I felt very sad, disappointed, and helpless for my aunt that she had been fooled by her own daughter. I knew my cousin took it and accused me of it because she was envious of me.

Two months after that incident, I moved to my mother's house. He would ask "why don't you step into my house anymore?" Too bad I didn't have a chance to tell my uncle the reason why.

"No reason, and I like to stay outside," I would respectfully say to him because I acknowledged the truth could hurt his feelings. He's deceased now, and he will always be in my heart next to my brother Xay.

6

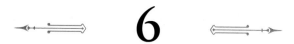

A year later, when I was in third grade, I met my cousin's friend at the Buddhist temple, and she told me my cousin was the one who took the money. She also told her not to tell my aunt about it. She continued, "Your cousin didn't want you to live with her family anymore, and she wanted her mom to kick you out. I'm sorry I lied for her, but she is my friend."

"It's okay because I know myself more than anybody else in this world. Thank you for telling me the truth." I also told her I would not stay in Thailand any longer.

My mother was a kind and generous person; she sacrificed herself for us. She left her hometown and her country again so she could come with us to the United States. All five children and parents moved to Ubon refugee camp in the middle of 1980, and we stayed at the camp for several months.

My family and I came to the USA in December of 1980—a total of twelve of my brothers and sisters came to the United States. My life was tough growing up and living in this country that I called home. We had to learn English fluently, and we had to adapt ourselves to a new climate. Because we came from a tropical climate, the snow in this States was new to all of us. We lived in a bad neighborhood. We were treated badly by the neighbors; many of them were prejudiced against us and discriminated us because my family and I looked different from them. We were new arrivals in the neighborhood.

Our parents were too old to find decent jobs to support us. There were six of us: my older brother Xay, an older sister, a younger brother, two younger sisters, and me. At first, we didn't have a car for our family. We commuted by city buses and walked by foot. Imagine walking in the snow for a couple miles in the winter. It was very complicated compared to the summer time. Sometimes our older sisters would come to pick up our mom to go shopping with them. We lived and grew up in bad neighborhoods.

We moved every time the landlord increased the house rent. We got our first family car when my brother Xay was in high school. He and my sister worked hard, and they gave our parents some of their money. I started fifth grade at Kenny Elementary. I loved that school very much. I had many wonderful teachers, and I met many friendly people there. I learned English pretty quickly and helped my parents by tutoring my youngest sister with her homework. I attended her conferences as well.

It was a nightmare for me while attending junior high school. Most of the students there were so prejudiced against Asian people, and I never felt safe at that school. I had to watch my back all the time when I walked by myself in the hallway. At the same time, I had been struggling with my life. I tried my best to study hard for my future. I used to have courage, self-respect, and ambition. Too much discrimination turned me into a person with low self-esteem. I got yelled at with racial slurs. "Chinese, Vietnamese, Japanese, go back to your country!" I was none of the above. This statement was one of their favorites. I ignored and walked away from those bullies many times for many years.

One time, I got tripped on the school bus by a bully for no reason. I went home and told my older sister Star about it. Thanks to Star, who knew how to fight, she settled the matter with her own hands. The bully learned the expensive lesson that day and became her friend after that.

The clinic and the convenience store were between one and two miles away from our house. We got there by foot. On the way there, we had to watch out for the bullies and be vigilant of the men who were intoxicated. They were usually around the sidewalk or at the park. Some days, we had to deal with more than one obstacle. Our mother told us, "Don't fight with them. Just ignore and walk away from them."

I remember one summer day I walked to the clinic by myself, and on the way home, I was surrounded by bullies. I was very frightened; I had a pathological fear. I took a big breath, and the first word that popped up in my mind at that moment was, "Run! Run! Run!" I decided to run for my life. Thank God for giving me all the strength to get away from them. They didn't have a chance to do anything to me because I ran faster than they did. I personally don't believe in physical fights; however, I don't mind fighting one-on-one to defend myself. On the other hand, most of the time, those bullies ganged up on those who are alone. To prevent all these troubles, we decided not to walk alone anymore.

The worst of the worst was when my mother was robbed at our front door. The unexpected happened to her again. It was a summer day. It was my mother and my younger brother's unlucky day to go grocery shopping. The bullies stopped them on the way home. They grabbed and tossed our groceries on the street. They attempted to hit my mother and my younger brother, who was about nine or ten years old at that time. Thank goodness, my brother was able to escape from them and was able to run home safely. There also was a Good Samaritan who warned those bullies from beating up my mom on the street. After they left the scene, our mom picked up our groceries from the street with hurt feelings and walked home. We were terrified when my brother ran home and told us about what happened, and we didn't have a chance to thank that Good Samaritan because by the time we got there, he was already gone.

I constantly had to deal with the bullies. On one incident, I was playing in the front yard by myself. Suddenly there was a bully approaching me with racial slurs again, and she was about to hit me, but this time I was ready for her. My instinct was telling me to fight her. I became very aggressive for the first time in my life, and I jumped at her before she even had a chance to fight back. I proved to her what's "Less talk, more actions" is. This person probably didn't realize that I had compiled all my strength to get ready and to be vigilant to defend myself from the bullies. They repeatedly abused us for many years, and many times, I had ignored, ran, or walked away from them. I had forgiven them for their bad behaviors. On the other hand, they thought I was a coward, and these bullies had made our lives a living hell.

The last incident that happened to me was when I was in high school. I had wanted to have a small garden, and one day, when I was busy digging in the dirt, I heard my neighbor yell at me, "Chinese, Japanese, go back to your country." I ignored her and kept working. She kept yelling at me for a few minutes; she didn't like my reaction. Then she decided to walk back inside her house.

A month later, I was very satisfied with my beautiful vegetables in the garden; I enjoyed watering them every day. One day, an unexpected thing happened to my garden. I was shocked and couldn't believe what I saw in front of me. Someone had destroyed most of my vegetables by stepping on them. "Why, why would they destroy them? They're not only mean to me; apparently they were being mean to my vegetables too," I whispered to myself. It was very hurtful and a burden, and I was very disappointed at my neighbors. I knew they did it, but I couldn't do anything about it. After that incident, I lost interest in gardening. At the same time, I promised myself, "One day I will move away from this city and live in a nice neighborhood so my children won't have to deal with the situation I have."

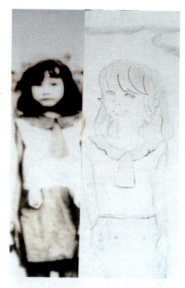

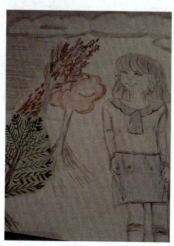

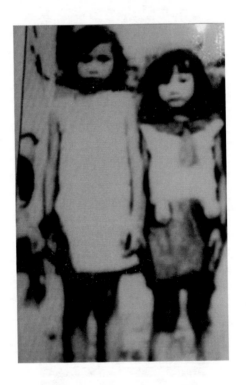

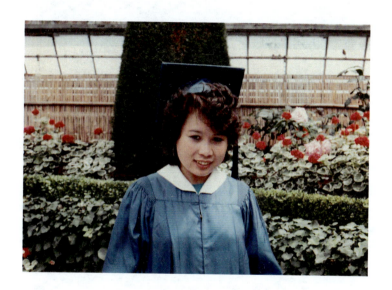

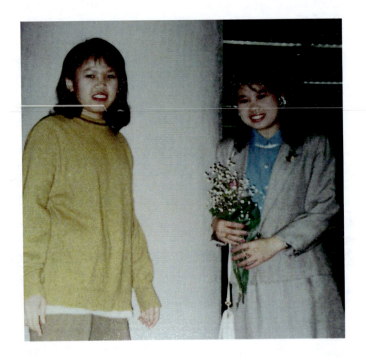

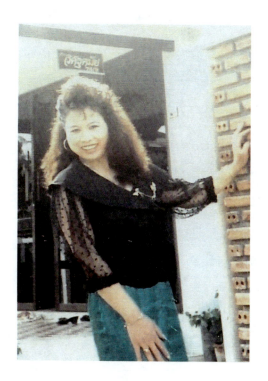

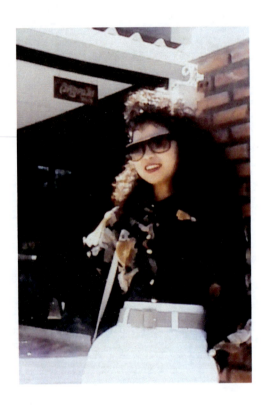

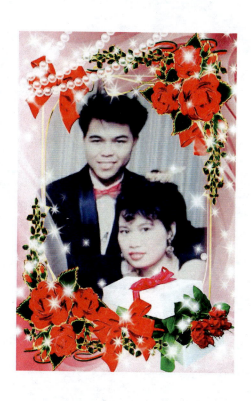

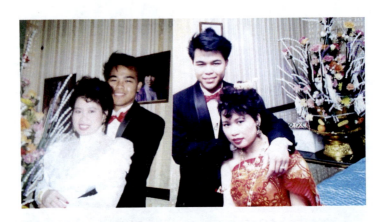

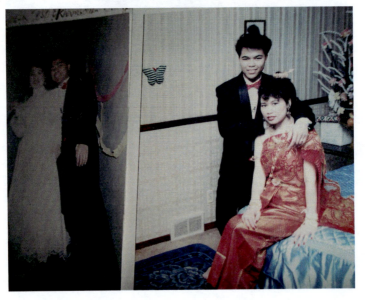

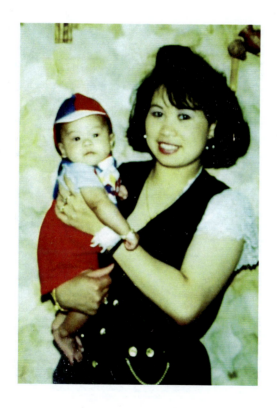

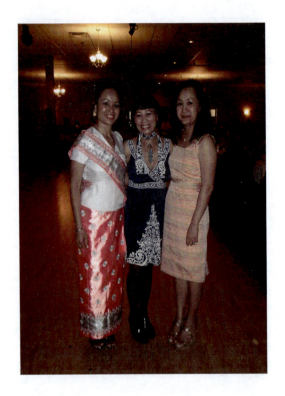

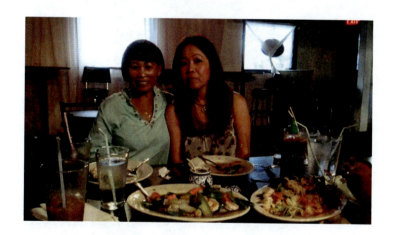

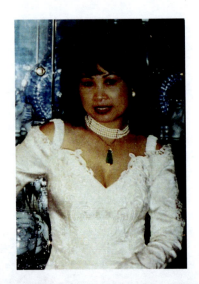

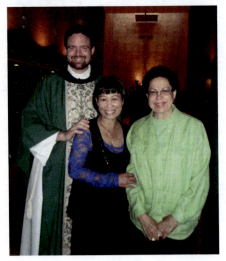

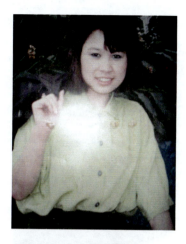

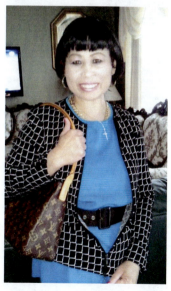

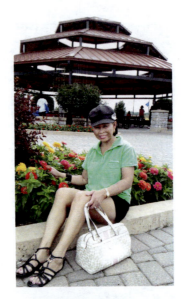

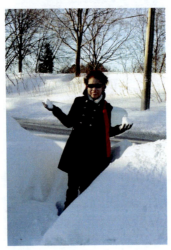

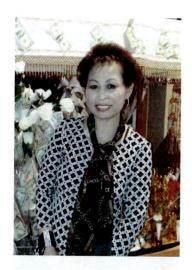

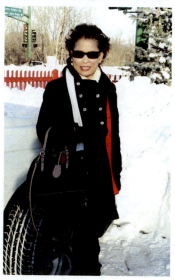

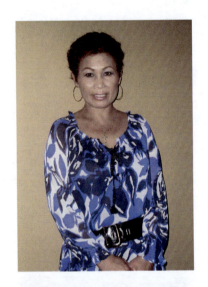

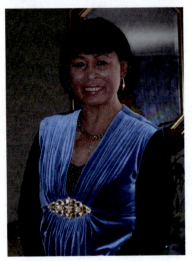

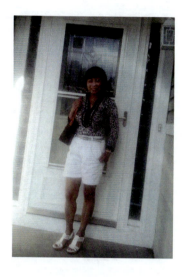

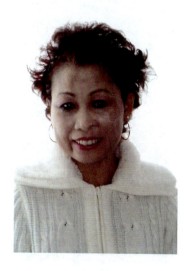

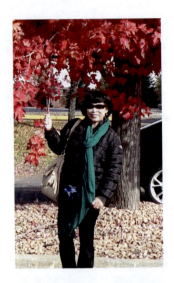

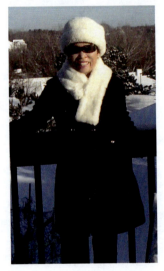

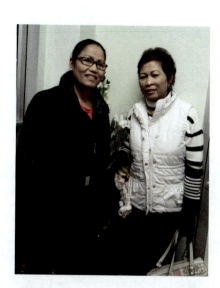

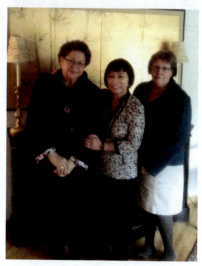

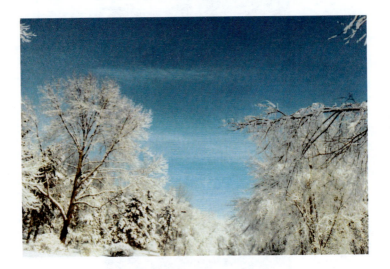

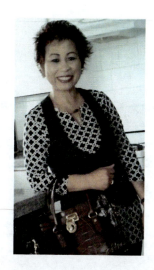

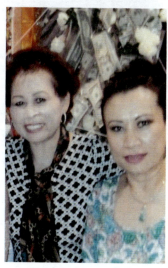

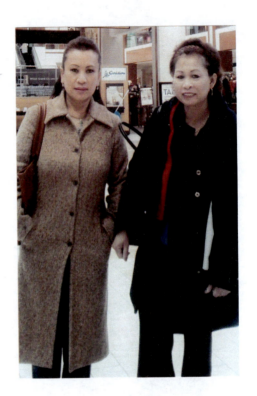

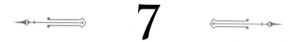

7

I started my first summer job after finishing 8th grade. I also worked during the weekends. Later on, I worked at the fast-food restaurant close to my house. I had a good time, and I enjoyed working there. Most importantly, I had a chance to work with a nice lady who took care of me like I was her own daughter. To the best of my knowledge, my parents tried their hardest raising us in the United States, especially because we were surrounded by many bad people. I respectfully say I'm grateful and honored, and I loved my parents unconditionally.

During my freshman year in high school, I met someone special at a party in Illinois. He was a nice person, but unfortunately, our relationship came to an end because of the long distance and we were too young to be a couple.

It was my sophomore year in high school when I met a significant person. He helped me get a part-time job at a restaurant on the weekends until I graduated from high school in 1987. I also came in second place in a two-year accounting program. Too bad there was only one scholarship for this program—no award for me.

One day, my telephone rang. I picked it up.

"Hi, can I speak to Khongmy Teso?" he said.

"Khongmy, speaking," I responded.

He gave me his name, and the company he worked for.

"How do you know me, and where did you get my number?" I asked.

"I found your name on the computer. I saw that you graduated with the highest score, for a minority student in accounting for 1987. He continued, "I am calling to ask if you would like you to come here for an orientation into an internship program, where you would work for our company, and we will pay for your continuing schooling."

I was very happy and proud of myself because a big corporation was interested in me, but I turned their offer down because of my low self-esteem and I didn't have a car to attend the orientation at the company.

I began to notice that my father had started to drink more and more. I'd never seen him drink like that before. He had become a totally different person from whom I remembered back in Laos. He probably felt bad about what we experienced here versus how we were raised as untouchable kids back in Laos. He couldn't do much about it because of the language barrier. It was tough for him living in the country we called the land of freedom and opportunities.

It was during my freshman year at the community college that my father got very ill, and I had to do my share taking care of him until he died in April of 1988.

"Can you look after your mother and your youngest sister for me when I'm gone?" he said to me on the night before he died. "I apologize for what I did to you emotionally."

I listened to him talk with tears in my eyes and cried with him. "It is okay. I forgive you. I understand you have too many children. Mom and you also tried your best to raise us here," I told him.

He said thank you to me and that he appreciated my kindness. It was the first and the last conversation and the best conversation I have ever had with him for the many years we had as father and daughter.

I decided to transfer from the community college to a technical college; I planned to pursue my goals later. I studied hard about America's constitutions and laws after I turned eighteen years old in September of 1987. I couldn't wait to take the citizenship test before the winter, and I passed it. I was very proud of myself and was very excited at that moment. On the form, I changed my name from Khongmy Teso to Anita Nina Teso because it was not my real name, but it was on the paper like that.

Of course, I officially became a naturalized citizen in 1988. They only charged me fifty dollar, but now it costs a lot more than that. I took *ani* from my Laotian name *Khongmani*, and *ta* from my Thai name *Nuntana*, and I combined them together to be called Anita. I did the same thing with my middle name.

My good friend Ketmani Kouancho had a huge impact in my life during my high school years at Edison High School. We had known each other since middle school. She had high self-esteem and was a confident and intelligent person. She encouraged me to take an English class with her, and she took me under her wing. She took me to a few entertainment places in the city and showed me around the cities in our state.

A couple of weeks after my father passed away, she came to pick me up at my house for the Laotian New Year's party at the university where she was attending school in 1988. She was in charge of the food, and her sister was in the fashion show.

The fashion show was very interesting, and her sister was very pretty, but I was unable to identify her partner because it was a little too dark at the fashion show. I turned to Ketmani and said, "Can you find somebody else to walk with your sister?"

"He is a student at the U," she replied.

Oops! I accidentally said that about my future husband!

Everything went great at the party, and I certainly enjoyed it very much. I loved hanging out with my good friend as well.

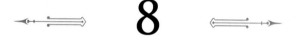

8

My mother became ill after she lost my dad. She missed him a lot; I noticed she listened to his favorite songs many times when she was alone. I went to school and worked part-time until I graduated. I left my house at 6:00 a.m. to catch a city bus to school. I walked several blocks from my school to the workplace after I finished with all of my classes. I worked as a data-entry operator, and my work schedule was 5:00 p.m. to 10:00 p.m. until I graduated from college. I graduated from the technical college and received a certificate for data-entry operator. I started working as a full-time employee for a good company in 1989.

It was a few months later when we all decided to move away from this terrible neighborhood to Richfield (suburb). Within a year of working, I was able to buy my first brand-new car in 1990.

My sister and I decided to take our mother to visit her family in Thailand in September of 1990. I was very excited to go back home, but everything didn't turn out the way I had pictured it.

We stayed at my uncle's house for a few weeks. I was very glad to see him once again. He was retired from work. I gave him some gifts as a way of expressing my gratitude to him for all the things he did for me when I was younger. Some of my cousins said I was more American than Thai. I didn't understand what they expected from me. I was just being myself. So I took it as a compliment. I was Asian American, bilingual, bicultural, bireligious (Buddhist and Christian). We stayed in Thailand for only six weeks. Someday I would like to take my family there again.

When I came back to the USA, I stayed in Modesto, California, for a year with my mother and my youngest sister. It took me only one week to find a job. I believe I was blessed. "What goes around comes around," as the saying goes.

Someone else who I appreciated very much for being so supportive was my brother-in-law. He and my sister let me borrow their car for one year without charging me for it.

My mother's condition had gotten better due to the nice weather in California, so we decided to return to Richfield in August of 1991. I was honored when my California boss mentioned to me on my last day of work, "Anita, I will rehire you anytime if you return to Modesto."

"Thank you very much," I respectfully said.

I returned to Richfield in August of 1991. I stayed with my oldest sister Diamond, the one who bought me those two dresses back in the old days. In November of 1991, my sister and I were invited to a Thanksgiving party. I was introduced to three good-looking young men, and the last one had a very attractive smile. He had darker skin, but honestly, I didn't pay much attention to that. I didn't realize he was the same person that I saw a few years earlier at the university. Was it a coincidence?

One day, in December of 1991, my sisters and I went to a Christmas party. At the party, there were the same three men I met at the Thanksgiving party. They came to ask us to dance for many songs until the band members took a break. Then my younger sister asked me to look around to see if I could find someone whom I would be interested in. So I looked around the room at all different faces, and I finally pointed at one man who was walking across the dance floor at that moment.

My younger sister May said, "Oh, gosh! That's Ken—he has been asking me to set up a blind date for you guys, but I ignored him. The first time he saw your picture with me at work, he seemed interested in you."

My older sister Star said, "That's Charlie—he told me to let him know when you came back home because he wanted to pick you up with me at the airport."

That was a coincidence; they were both talking about the same person who went by two different names! When the party was over, Charlie and two of his friends walked us out to the car and said they would give us a call after the New Year.

On the second day of 1992, I received a telephone call from Charlie and many calls after that. He seemed to be a nice guy and was also the type of person who would not take no for an answer. I guess destiny had brought us together. It must have been love at first sight for him.

"No, I'm too busy." I refused him a couple times, but he continued calling me anyway.

"We can have the four of us go out for dinner!" he said.

"Okay!" I said.

We double-dated with my older sister and his friend. Once I got to know him, he was not bad. He sincerely cared for my mother. Because of her health issues, I had to take her to many doctor appointments, and he went with me. On one visit to a doctor, Mom got bad news. "Your mom will either be blind or pass away in 1993," the doctor said.

He seemed to be a kind person, a gentleman. He fascinated me with his charm and his attractive smile. I have to admit that it was hard not to immediately fall in love with a person who has a good sense of humor like him. That was how he won my heart in such a short period of time. We dated for a few months, and our love eventually grew so strong that he proposed marriage.

"Will you marry me?" he asked me with his attractive smile.

He took my breath away with his proposal; at that moment, I felt very happy, like the whole world was all mine. "Yes, yes!" I responded quickly.

My heart was pounding even after saying yes. I felt my heart swell up inside me, and it flooded with pure happiness. It was the most exciting moment of my life.

I did experience mixed emotions that day. Part of it was my concern for my mother's health conditions, whom I was taking care of at the time. Another part was my readiness to begin my adult life. I come from a very strict culture and family that require single women to stay with their parents or with older brothers or sisters.

My husband and I got married on December 23, 1992. We went to the courthouse and had a justice of the peace marry us. He said, "You guys are a cute couple and very young to get married. I won't charge you for my service, but you have to pay for the paperwork."

"Thank you very much, sir, for an early Christmas present," I said.

"You're welcome!" he responded with a big smile on his face.

After that, we had a wedding on December 26, 1992, and Charlie gave me a diamond ring, gold, and money as dowry. Then I finally moved out from my sister's house to our apartment and so began our new family together.

Happily, our mom beat the odds—she's still alive until August 26, 2013.

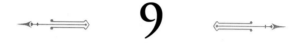

9

Just when I'd started having a happy life with my family, life was unfair to me once again. One day, I did not feel well, so my husband took me to see a doctor. She gave us good and bad news at the same time. She stated that I was a couple of months pregnant, but I had a bladder infection and hypertension, and soon after that I was diagnosed with IgA nephropathy. My kidney was functioning about 60 to 70 percent at that time. This time, I had to fight with my illness.

I prayed for a healthy baby. I had morning sickness all day long for many months; I was unable to eat much of anything, but I forced myself to eat each time. I was usually dehydrated and had to go to a clinic for an IV a couple of times. The doctor gave me medications to control the high-blood pressure. I was very lucky that my husband helped me around the house. He did a marvelous job. I was very grateful that we supported and loved each other.

My husband and I were expecting a baby boy. He was born in May of 1993. My husband took care of our son for three months before he returned to work. I was very fortunate to have a helper like him. He was a wonderful husband and a wonderful father as well.

Motherhood was very challenging for me when I returned to work after three months of maternity leave. Being a full-time mother and full-time employee plus having health problems made my daily life very difficult, but I didn't give up. Luckily, we were able to manage it. In one year we had saved up enough money to buy our first house in a nice city and a good neighborhood.

A few months later, I had a kidney biopsy and discovered that I had kidney stones that needed to be removed from both of my kidneys. One-day surgery was required. I felt a little better after the procedure.

I had kidney failure toward the end of 1997. This time I would have to fight for my life once again. I started my first hemodialysis treatments. These treatments were on Mondays, Wednesdays, and Fridays—three hours each time—for two and a half years. During dialysis, I sometimes experienced body cramps, high- or low-blood pressure, low pulse, and more. I was thankful for hemodialysis treatments and the staff at the dialysis unit, though, for saving my life.

It was in the summer, sometime after 5:30 p.m., and I was on my way to the dialysis unit when suddenly my body became stiff. That meant I had high potassium in my system, which can cause death. I prayed for a miracle to protect me from a car accident. I was on a very busy Highway 169 during rush hour. I was blessed again. I was able to get to the parking lot without any accident. I got out of the car and then was standing by the car because I was unable to move. After a few minutes, an unknown lady stopped after several other people had passed by me. This wonderful lady noticed that I was in distress and asked, "Do you need help? Where do you want me to take you to?"

I nodded my head, and I tried to roll my eyes to my left arm so she would see the arteriovenous graft on my left arm. After she saw that, surprisingly, she knew where to take me right away.

"The reason I knew where to take you is because my mother-in-law used to have this problem. She has since passed away. You'll be fine because you are young," she told me on the way to the dialysis unit. I only looked at her because I couldn't talk or move my body at that time. She got a wheelchair and took me to the dialysis unit and shouted, "She needs help!"

They rushed to get me on the machine. After that, the registration nurse said to me, "Anita, you have high potassium, and you're about one minute away from having a heart attack or stroke."

I stared silently at them. I was very fortunate and thankful for that wonderful lady who saved my life that day.

Due to the dialysis treatments, I lost about 80 percent of my hair. I ended up shaving it each time it occurred. I experienced a few symptoms, such as tightness on my skull. It was painful, and I felt uncomfortable for a few days before hair began to fall out. As a result, I had to wear a wig when going out in public. At first, I didn't like to wear a wig because it did not feel comfortable, but after a while, I got used to it. Wearing a wig gave me a different look, and I liked it.

A couple times it happened, I went to see doctors, but they came up with nothing because all the lab work was negative. I tried my best to endure and held my head up high like nothing had happened even though sometimes I would feel sad and burdened inside. I tried to hide it from everybody. I always had a big smile on my face when I went out with my family and friends, but nobody knew what I felt inside.

It wasn't easy for me to overcome my own emotional distress. I thank God for sending a young lady who saved my life. I was inspired by this young lady whom I met only one time at the dialysis unit around 1998–1999. I had noticed her health condition and felt sorry for her. This helped me gain more self-confidence, and it certainly helped me to clear up my mind as I had been questioning to myself, "Should I leave or stay with my only child?" After that, I decided not to give up on life, and I would fight to stay alive.

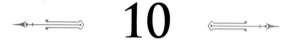

10

I started working for a big company in 1992 as an office clerk. Six months later, I got a job offer as department coordinator, and after that, I worked as an accounting clerk (accounts receivable) with high recommendation within the same company. I was lucky enough to have the opportunity to work with many great people.

The conflicts at work created a big impact in my daily life. When one co-worker joined our department, I trained her and treated her with respect even though she was so indifferent to me. I didn't mind working with her until one morning when I came to work after being absent. She asked me why I was absent, and I replied, "I didn't feel well and my son was sick too."

I felt hurt and disappointed at the way she said this to me and how she compared herself to my situation. I worked full-time, had health problems, and also had a baby who was sick almost every month until he was five years old. I was overwhelmed and in distress. It wasn't easy for me to overcome these obstacles. At the time, I was fighting emotional stress and peer pressure at work. I forced myself to become a stronger person, and I've never given up on life.

I went to see my favorite co-worker for comfort, and I told her about the incident.

"Anita, you are too nice, You can't respect everybody. You only treat people the way you want to be treated, but you have to learn how to defend yourself," she reminded me. I have remembered her statement ever since.

A year later, when my health condition got worse, I decided to take long-term disability. After that, I decided to resign from the company. It was about a year later when my health condition got better, so I went back to apply for an accounting-clerk position within the same company but in a different department, and I was hired.

The new me was a little bit different than the old me—I had become more Americanized. My culture growing up was quite the opposite of the American culture, and I had started to adopt more of the American ways. I was raised to be humble, observable, and a respectful person. I was so fortunate there were kind and generous bosses who gave me opportunities and who believed in my work. I worked very hard and had satisfied my bosses with my work performance. They both realized I had tried my best to work for them even though I had to go to the dialysis unit three times per week after work. Thank God for their help and support. I very much appreciated their kindness. I also believed in the virtue of faith.

There is a very good phrase that I go by: "What goes around comes around," which is the idea of karma. I believe it really exists. About a year later, I ran into someone from my past, and I was glad to see her. She was a wonderful person who treated me with respect through my difficult times during pregnancy.

"Anita, I wanted to apologize to you about what I said to you," she said.

"No, it is okay!" I replied.

"It is not okay, Anita." She looked at me.

She didn't know I had forgiven her a long time ago because she used to be very nice and kind to me, and I still like her.

One afternoon I heard someone calling my name from behind. I turned around to see who it was. She approached me and said, "Anita, do you remember me?"

I hardly recognized her. "Oh yeah!" I said.

She told me about what had happened to her lately, and a few minutes later, we both said good-bye to each other. She was my former coworker. I certainly hoped the best for her because she went through a lot after I left that department, according to what she had just told me. Plus I had moved on with my life, and I would never step on or take advantage of a sick person like someone did to me.

A few months after that incident, I ran into a third person from my past in the cafeteria. She looked at me. "Anita, I wanted to apologize to you about what I said to you before," she said.

"No, it is okay. You did what you had to do," I said.

She stared at me in the eyes and continued to talk. "Anita, I know how hard it is coming to work when you have a baby and when you're having health problems too."

I was glad that she realized after all. I had forgiven her a long time ago. I had learned from it. I became a stronger person, and I became a fighter because of these people.

11

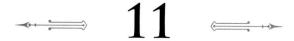

I n the middle of 2000, I saw a familiar face, and I approached this nice lady. "Are you a teacher?" I asked.

"Yes, and I'm still teaching sixth grade students at Kenwood Elementary School. Why are you asking me that?" she responded.

"You look like my sixth grade teacher from Kenny Elementary School."

Mrs. Lynne Raphael and I were reunited, and we kept seeing each other weekly. I had respected my former teacher because she and Mrs. Cecelia Kirihara, my ESL teachers from fifth and sixth grade, impressed me with good memories before I moved on to junior high school. I enjoyed every time we talked, and I was very glad to see she was all right to this day. I honestly have respect for Lynne and consider her as my second mother because she is a wonderful person.

It was November 30, 2000, while I was still at the dialysis unit, when I received a telephone call from the transplant coordinator. This was the third call I had received from them.

"Is this Anita? You need to go to the hospital right after dialysis, okay?"

"Okay, I will be there as soon as possible," I responded.

My husband and I went to the hospital after we came home to see our son. When we got to the hospital, they put us in the small waiting room. I prayed and anxiously waited for good news; hopefully, it would be a perfect match this time. "Yes, the third time is a lucky charm," I said.

It was my early Christmas present. I got a kidney transplant in the early morning of December 1, 2000. It was a 99.9 percent match. Before they delivered me to a surgery room, my doctor told me it would take at least two days for the kidney to kick in. I prayed for my new kidney to kick in right away, and there was a miracle once again. When I woke up, I discovered that the doctor was wrong about that. I was so delighted and excited, and I couldn't wait to go home to see my family. The doctor told me to go home on the third day of hospitalization. Oh, I was very satisfied with my kidney-transplant surgeon at that hospital. He had done a marvelous job for me.

The doctor had given me the antirejection drugs, and I had been taking higher doses because I had received a new kidney from a cadaver (dead donor). Otherwise, my body would reject the new kidney eventually. It was different from the people who had received a new kidney from a living donor. I was discharged from the hospital on the evening of the third day after the transplant, but some of the other patients stayed for a week or more at that time.

Before I left the building, I noticed that I had weird symptoms. I requested a doctor to have the blood work done to make sure I could still go home. I was afraid to go only halfway and have to come back again. Less than an hour later, the results came.

"You are right about it. You are having a reaction to the antirejection drugs. It has destroyed your kidney function."

I was so disappointed after the doctor told me the bad news. I had a very good kidney, but it only stayed with me for three days.

It was a nightmare; I had been through a lot for the new kidney to regain its functions. I'd been treated for rejection, and I had a high temperature—up to 102 degrees—every time they injected the medicine to treat the transplanted kidney so it would function again. Thanks for the ice packs they provided me each time.

I had kidney biopsies many times both by my own doctor and by a resident. I stayed in the hospital until December 31, 2000. That meant I was in the hospital exactly for one month. Before I left the hospital, they recommended a brand-new medicine. I would be the first person taking this medicine from their hospital. I decided to take the risk. Despite all the troubles, the doctor told me that a new kidney would function only four to five years.

I went home with the second antirejection drug. From January until the middle of March 2001, I was taking the new drug. I went to the hospital to have the blood work done weekly, and basically, they told me everything was fine. Until one day, they told me not to go there anymore. I needed to go to the convenient clinic instead, and I did what they had told me to do in the following week. I understood that the doctors did their best to care for me. The word *reaction* made me feel uncomfortable and scared. I believe it was on March 15, 2001, when I received a telephone call stating that I had to be admitted to the hospital because the new medicine had destroyed my plasma. I felt sick to my stomach to hear bad news like that.

"Who gave it to you and for how long have you been taking it?" my new doctor asked me.

I told my doctor about who had given me the medicine and for how long I had been taking it. This time I was under the care of a different doctor and at a different hospital. I was hospitalized for ten days. I continued with plasmapheresis (plasma exchange) as an outpatient more than a month. Each treatment would run for three hours, and I would be extremely tired after the treatment each time. I had to rest in the lounge for at least half an hour in order for me to be able to drive myself home from a big city to the suburb.

I repeated the weekly process over and over again until one day, right before I was attached to the machine, I was informed by the technician that my plasma was normal according to the blood work. However, my schedule required one more week, then I'd be done with the treatments. I tried to convince my doctor to discontinue the treatments, but I was unsuccessful. Poor Anita had to continue the treatments for another week. When I'd been on the machine for about one hour, I started to have a very bad reaction. I felt like I was going to die; however, I told myself to focus, to be vigilant, and to fight for my life at all times. I was in critical condition, and I couldn't respond to my doctor. After that, they delivered me to the emergency room and less than one hour later, I was doing fine.

When the registration representative was entering my information, I stopped her right away and said, "I don't want to stay overnight here."

"I will call your doctor about it," she said.

I personally had experienced and learned from my own body about the symptoms. A few minutes later, my doctor arrived, and I was able to convince her to discharge me from the emergency room that night.

"If you have any symptoms, then call 911," she said.

"Nothing will happen to me. You are my doctor, and I am supposed to listen to you, but if you would have listened to me at the first time, none of this would have happened to me." I proudly had defended myself by saying it to her, and I got it out from my chest. At the same time, I didn't hear any comments from her. After that we both looked at each other silently before she left the room.

"Bye-bye!" she said.

"Bye-bye!" I responded.

Finally, I was able to go home and never continued the treatment again.

The treatment was very difficult and uncontestable. I didn't attempt any lawsuits against the doctors or the hospitals for the pain and suffering I went through. I had forgiven them and believed that it was just a human error. Because of reaction, my life would never be the same. After going back to work, I seemed to have trouble with memory a little bit. I was under a lot of stress at work, and my kidney function got worse, so I decided to resign from the accounting department, and my career was coming to an end with this good company in 2004.

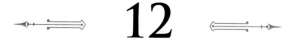

12

It seemed like one thing led to another. This time I had to fight with the pain on the left side of my face. It was just a few months after I was discharged from the hospital in 2001. I had the worst shingles on the left side of my face because of my weakened immune system. It was the worst of the worst shingles I had ever imagined. It looked horrible, and it was very uncomfortable and painful. I looked at myself in the mirror, and I couldn't believe what I saw on my face. I went to see a doctor two times. The second time I went to a different doctor, and he prescribed medicine for me to take. I suffered for many months before it disappeared from my face, but I suffered for many years from the pain.

The shingles left scars on my face, and as a result of it, the scar tissue was blocking my left nostril. It was too complicated to come up with a procedure to make it work and have it look normal. That's what I was told by two doctors from two different hospitals. I honestly didn't feel comfortable to have the surgery. Hopefully someday I will be able to have cosmetic surgery done to remove the scar tissue from my left nostril. To this day, it is still hard to breathe because of my left nostril. Hopefully my wishes will come true someday.

After I'd recovered from the kidney transplant and the shingles, my boss was kind enough to offer me a new position working in the general-ledger department full time. Later on I would be working four hours in the general ledger and four hours in the payroll department each day. However, I only started in general ledger for a few months when I received bad news that payroll would be moving to a different state. Obviously, I had a potential employment opportunity to return to work in the accounts-receivable department again, but it would be under a new supervisor.

When I returned to the department, I noticed that I would be working with a new group of people. I was fine with this except for the supervisor. She was indifferent, and there was no connection between us whatsoever. I tried very hard to win her heart by my work performance, but I had to give it up because of my poor health. The treatment caused much suffering and was uncontestable. Because of reaction, my life would never be the same. I was under a lot of stress at work, and my kidney function got worse. I decided to resign from the company again even though I had learned and gained a lot of knowledge from this company. I honestly appreciated most of the people that I met, especially those people who believed in me and those who supported me while I was working for them.

My kidney only worked for a little over four years and then failed on me. I had to have it removed. I returned to the dialysis unit in 2004 for a second time, and I received dialysis at a unit close by my house. Everything was going fine until one day I had a weird symptom—diarrhea—during dialysis. I lost more than five pounds because of it. They were afraid that I might have parasites. An esophagogastroduodenoscopy (EGD), a bone-marrow biopsy, and other tests were required. The bone-marrow biopsy was the most painful of all procedures I'd done in the summer.

All the tests came back negative, and I called my doctor. "Maybe I was allergic to the reused dialyzer and can I use a brand-new one instead?" He agreed with me right away and ordered the registered nurse to use the brand-new dialyzer for me. As a result, I never had diarrhea anymore, and I was right about it too.

I appreciated my nephrologist for taking good care of me. I have used his services since 1993, and I'm very satisfied. I will recommend him to everyone I know because he is a good doctor.

I decided to go visit my sister in California for two weeks. While there, I went to a dialysis unit near her house. I was satisfied with most of the staff and their services. Overall, hemodialysis is good for me; it is a lifesaver. I'm so grateful and appreciative to all of the staff at the dialysis unit where I'm at now for taking good care of me for all these years. I thank God that we have dialysis units around the United States.

I've been through a lot of pain (survived three car accidents in my life) especially that it is uncomfortable for me to be on a chair for three hours each time with back pain during dialysis treatments. I went to dialysis every Monday, Wednesday, and Friday every week. At first, I had treatment with the chiropractor on Tuesday and Thursday for many weeks, and then after that it was once every two weeks, and later it was once a month for over a year. Thank God it is over! It was time-consuming, and it took a long time for me to overcome the pain, but I'm okay now.

My good friend Ketmani from high school and I were reunited at her sister's house around the summer of 2005. I saw my husband and her sister having a conversation. I approached both of them and introduced my husband to her.

"We already know each other," they responded about the same time.

I turned to Ketmani's sister and said, "Don't tell me that he is the same person who walked with you that day at the U."

She responded by nodding her head with a big smile.

I looked at them at the same time. I realized he was the same man who was in the fashion show with her that night back in the old days. I was surprised, and I smiled at both of them, a little embarrassed because I never thought in a million years that my husband was the same man I saw during the fashion show that night at the university in April of 1988. Wow! I assumed he was a gift from God, sending him to love, to support, and to take good care of me while I was struggling with my health.

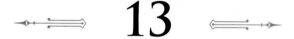

13

I had been living my life as normal as possible and staying as persistent as I could until one summer day, I had to go to the emergency room with my son because I didn't feel good. They admitted me to the hospital on July 19, 2010. I was transferred to a single room upstairs because I had high-blood pressure, heartburn, and palpitations. Later they found I had pneumonia.

A strange thing happened to me while I was in the hospital that time. Some people will believe me, and some people will not. Ever since that incident occurred, I've been wondering and trying to remember what really happened to me back in July of 2010.

A few weeks ago, I called my younger sister and asked her to fill in with more details about the whole thing because she was there when it happened to me.

"I don't feel comfortable telling you all the details," she honestly said.

"Okay," I said.

I vividly remembered that both of my parents strongly believed in spiritual stuff, and I totally believed there were clean and unclean spirits out there and that anything is possible in this world.

"Did you have a conversation with a nurse when you came to visit me for the first time? When was I acting strange to you? When did you come to see me?" I asked her.

"Yes, I talked to a nurse. You were acting strange, and I came to visit you in the evening," she told me.

"What! In the evening?" I was shocked.

My sister also mentioned she knew that I wasn't myself at that time, and it looked like someone else was inside of me because I never talked and acted like that in my entire life.

I was in critical condition. I was put through a lot of tests and was treated with medications to control the complication. I was admitted to a telemetry unit on a nitroglycerin infusion due to a significantly elevated blood pressure of 246/123 at one point. But I was still okay—no heart attack or stroke; maybe I was lucky this time. Normally, for most people, a blood pressure that high would cause a stroke or a heart attack. The doctor ordered six kinds of blood-pressure medication for me to take, and as a result, my blood pressure was better, but there was no satisfaction yet.

When I saw the room for the first time, I mentioned to my husband how much I liked the room because it was light and airy. It was till daylight, though, around 5:30 p.m. when we came in. For the first couple days, I turned all the lights on at night, including the restroom's lights, and I kept my front door open all the time. I felt like there was something strange in that room, especially at night.

"Anita, no wonder you can't sleep. You have all the lights on. Let me turn off some of them," a nurse mentioned to me on one occasion.

"Okay, go ahead," I replied.

She turned off the lights, including the one in the rest room. She dimmed a light above my head so it would help me to fall asleep easier.

"Don't close the door!" I told her.

"Why?" she questioned me.

"I'm scared of the dark," I replied. After that, I dimmed the light above my head and turned off all the lights in my room like she had done.

On the third day, my doctor told me I could go home around noon after finishing dialysis. My appointment was around 7:00 or 7:30 a.m. For some reason, I couldn't sleep that night. I had the television on the Gospel Channel too. Perhaps I was too anxious and excited to go home. I tried my best to fall asleep, but I did not succeed. I looked up at the clock across from my bed, and it was 4:15 a.m.

I tried for the second time to sleep, but I had closed my eyes for only a few moments when I heard a noise from an object that hit the edge of my bed. It felt like some object hit me on the right side of my face. I immediately opened my eyes in fear and discovered that it was a tissue box. I was very scared and frightened. I quickly pressed the nurse button right away. A few minutes later, a nurse came in the room.

"Do you need some help? How can I help you?" she asked.

"No, I just want to know who threw the tissue box at me," I responded.

"Nobody is in your room. Do you want me to put it away for you?"

"Okay," I said.

I handed it to her, and she put it away for me. Then she turned to leave. I turned my face toward the door so I could see her walking out of my room. At that moment, I saw a dark form and felt that something or someone was watching me from the front of my bed. I was going to yell to the nurse for help, but it was too late. The dark presence suddenly moved toward me and hit me on my chest very hard, and the upper part of my body jerked off from the bed. After that, it either knocked me out or I blacked out, and I thought my life was over at that time.

I didn't remember what really happened after that, except that I had made a telephone call to my younger sister and her friend. Unfortunately, I couldn't remember all the conversation. That was the last time I remembered what was going on until I overheard a conversation between a nurse and my younger sister.

"What did Anita say to you before all this happened?" the nurse asked my younger sister. Someone else had mentioned that I had been watching the Gospel Channel at night. I could hear things, but I couldn't move or open my eyes.

It was probably a few minutes later that I was able to open my eyes and sit down on my bed. I realized that I was still alive—except there was something wrong with me. I was aware of what was going on the whole time. But I it find difficult to describe the feelings at that time. I was confused; it felt like something was present inside of me, especially on my chest. I wasn't myself. I was also aware that I was not the person who did the talking most of the time.

"Hi, Anita," greeted a lady who was walking in the hallway. She was probably a nurse or a nurse's assistant working that day.

"I am not Anita…I'm Anita's father, and I came to protect her!" a mysterious voice replied.

This was part of what I heard, and I was confused as there wasn't anyone in my room but me. I thought to myself, *Why am I hearing stuff like that? I know I did not say that.*

I was visited by the psychologist a few times, and he did some tests on me.

"You have a good memory!" he said to me twice during the tests because I passed all of his tests.

"Do you believe in spirits?" the mysterious voice said.

"Silence! Is it what you do to Anita?" the psychologist asked.

"You have to discharge Anita, and I'll leave her body alone, and I'll go home," the mysterious voice continued.

"Where is your home?" the psychologist questioned.

I heard the mysterious voice say, "Heaven!" He kept saying to both male and female psychologists that he was my father.

"We can't let Anita go home yet until her voice is clear and normal," the male psychologist said.

I recognized he came with his female partner a few times, and I realized the whole time that it wasn't really me who was talking to them. At the same time, I was questioning myself too. Why was I unable to say things that I wanted to say? I felt like something was taking charge of my body.

Many hours later, someone put in the order that I could go home the next morning after dialysis. The next day, my blood pressure became satisfactory about 20 minutes after the dialysis. Shortly afterward, I felt like the "something" that had overtaken my body was gone from my chest. I felt like I was being myself once again, but my eyes were very tired. When the nurse came into my room, I told her right away.

"I am myself now!" I said with a happy face.

"Let me take your blood pressure now," she said with smile.

After that, she was surprised because my blood pressure was very good (119/74). "Yes, you are. And look, your blood pressure is normal now," she said with a happy face.

"Yes!" I responded.

"I will let the doctors know about it," she said.

Later on, she went through all the medications with me as well as other documents. After that, I was discharged. I went home with six kinds of blood-pressure medication to take.

Several months after that incident, in 2011, my youngest sister opened up a little bit more, sharing details with me about the whole scary and strange experience that she had while I was in the hospital.

"When did you have a conversation with the nurse?" I asked.

"It was the evening of that day," she said.

"Oh, my goodness, had it been that long?" I asked. That meant I was knocked out or had blacked out and didn't remember anything from about 4:30 a.m. until the evening.

Overall, I realized and totally understood what really happened to me. It might sound weird or strange to many people who don't believe that spirits exist, unless you have experienced it yourself. On the other hand, for those people who believe that spirits do exist, they obviously had found the answer a while ago.

I was cured from a minor pneumonia before being discharged from the hospital. According to the discharge summaries on July 28, 2010, it stated that during the last three days of my stay in the hospital, I had developed "psychosis of questionable etiology" and the work-up was negative. Psychiatry was consulted, no medications were given, and I reverted back to baseline mental status before discharge.

There was a reason why my sister initially refused to tell me more about what actually happened to me because one strange thing had happened to her too. But she is now willing to tell me. One day, while she was talking to me on the telephone, I was not being myself. After she hung up the phone, she received a mysterious text message from an unknown number, saying,

> Anita O, blond hair, a singer, December 31, 1969,
> Not yet!

There was one creepier thing that I need to tell. The caller ID numbers that showed on her cellular phone belonged to my room at the hospital. She was so terrified that she dropped her telephone on the floor. She remembered that the conversation with me started out good, but then it seemed like another person was talking, and it scared her. It took her several months after the incident to tell me about what she had experienced while I was in the hospital for those nine days.

"Anita, when is your birthday?" she questioned.

"September 2, 1969. Why?"

"Who is Anita with a last name that starts with *O*, December 31, 1969?" she asked.

"I don't know. Only the name and the year match mine," I responded.

This is my conclusion to the best of my knowledge. The voice that I heard most of the time, I believe, was a good spirit. He indicated himself as my father, and he could be my dad coming to protect me from that mysterious dark force. Perhaps he just wanted to make sure that I would get out of the room and the hospital safely. The mysterious force could have been another Anita—Anita O—with a birthday of December 31, 1969, who might have stayed in that room or in the hospital.

I am not surprised if some doctors believed the reasons I had been acting out like that were because of my history, the medication I'd taken, or because I had very high-blood pressure for days. Everything that has happened is possible in this world! When you don't experience it, it doesn't mean that it does not exist. I just wanted to share about what I experienced while I was in the hospital. It really happened to me, even though it might be beyond belief to some people.

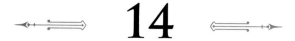

14

My troubles were not over yet! It was a Sunday evening, and I had eaten too many of the tomatoes from my garden. Too many tomatoes meant too much potassium, and too much potassium can cause death. My risks as a kidney patient are cardiovascular disease, bone health, immune-system function, depression, cancer, fluid retention, and polypharmacy (use of multiple medications).

Early Monday morning on August 9, 2010, before 1:00 a.m., I discovered some weird symptoms—shortness of breath, diarrhea, and vomiting many times. I told my son to telephone my husband to come home from work. About an hour later, he showed up. He asked me about my symptoms, and then he called 911 for the ambulance to take me to the hospital as I couldn't handle it any longer. A few minutes later, they came into our house. One paramedic grabbed my right arm and said, "I can't feel her pulse." When I heard that, I turned and looked at my husband right away. I discovered that he was watching me helplessly behind the paramedic crew.

My eyes closed automatically; they laid me down on the floor, and I started to pray for a miracle. "My Lord, please be with me, and don't let my soul leave my body. I pray in the name of Jesus Christ, Amen." Amazingly, I was able to hear what was going on the whole time. I told myself to stay focused, and it proved to me that I was still alive. They had to do an automated external defibrillator (AED) procedure on me to boost up my heart rate for a while.

"Ouch…ouch…ouch!" I kept complaining to them.

"I know, I know, it's painful, but just hang in there, okay?" somebody said to me. It was one of the paramedics who responded to me. It was a very painful procedure. It took them awhile before they stopped.

"We have her pulse now!" he said.

After that, they put me inside the ambulance. I heard the paramedic crew member ask, "What hospital does Anita usually go to?"

My husband told him the name of the hospital in South Minneapolis. "No, we cannot take her there because she is not going to make it. We have to take her to the nearest hospital," he said impatiently.

I was knocked out, and I didn't hear anything after that. Later, when I woke up, I realized that I was inside the ICU.

According to the clock on the wall across from me, it was around 3:00 a.m.

"I have high potassium from eating too many tomatoes, and it just needs to be dialyzed from my system," I mentioned to the nurse.

"We are getting a machine right now," he told me with a smile.

I fainted after that. When I next woke up, it was 5:00 p.m.

"You are waking up now. We are going to move you to a regular room," the nurse said.

Then they moved me to the regular room. I was in the intensive care unit for more than twelve hours. This was the second time I had high potassium, and both times it almost cost me my life. From now on, I would have to be vigilant because I might not be so lucky the next time. I am thankful to the paramedic team for saving my life that early morning and also the good doctors for saving my life at this hospital.

A good young doctor had told me that I was very lucky that day. "Don't do it again, okay?" he told me with a smile.

I didn't say anything, just responded by giving him a big smile instead.

I recently told a lady about this incident. She stated that most people she talked to had gone through the same situation as me. They told her that they were standing and watching the people working on their bodies. To me, it seemed like their souls had already left their bodies. But not mine—praise to the Lord and thank God for the miracle! As I recall, I probably was in the ICU more than three times in my life so far. Each of those times, the doctors had informed my family to come to the hospital since I was in critical condition and had a poor chance of survival, but I survived every time when it happened because I had a strong faith in God. Jesus has been my salvation.

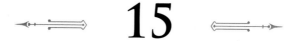

15

I love the United States of America—the third country that I have called home—but I will never forget about Laos and Thailand. I am very proud of my four nephews who joined the US Marines, the US Army, and the US Coast Guard to fight and protect this country.

It was a few years ago that I had an opportunity to welcome four soldiers into my home for a week. One of them was my nephew from California, who wanted to visit my family before he took off from Wisconsin to his destination. I knew my nephew was a fighter, and this was his second or third time going back to Iraq.

"Hi! Welcome to our home!" I greeted them.

"Thank you!" they responded.

They all were very young and very strong men. We were so delighted to see them, and we supported our soldiers. We enjoyed having barbecues with them in our backyard, and we also went out to eat with them while they were staying with us.

It's a fact of life: when you start with saying hi, you will always end up with saying good-bye. That day came, and we all said it to each other. Of course, we wished them the best of luck, and we wished them to return home safely and as soon as possible. I am very proud of my nephews, not only because they were born in the United States of America, but also because they have the opportunity to fight and protect it too. It's just like I am always proud to tell people that I come from a military family. Oh yes, I said that indeed.

I wish my dad were here. He would be very proud of his grandchildren, who were born in the freedom country, and most of them turned out okay.

16

I believe that faith and destiny brought my husband and me together. He is a wonderful man who has stood by me through everything. I have enjoyed every moment I've had with my son too—he is my life and my soul. My husband is my soul mate. Both of them have filled my life with happiness and made me feel life is worth living.

Many men and women have said to me, "You are very lucky that your husband is a kind and wonderful person. Most men would leave you right after they find out that you are sick," they said.

"Yes, I am, but we were born for each other!" I responded with a smile to the last man who said this to me.

On many occasions, I would go home and cry after hearing this statement from people. These people probably didn't know that it was not an appropriate thing to say to a sick person like me—or to anybody at all—because it is very hurtful and discouraging. My husband knew every time it occurred because I would keep tossing and weeping in bed.

"Don't care about what people have said to you," he said. "Let it go in one ear and out the other. Don't let it bother you too much. Why are you caring? Just focus on your health; take good care of yourself so you can stay with your son and husband."

"It's easier said than done," I said sadly.

From time to time, I had to learn to forgive, be strong, overcome, and handle all types of people and obstacles—I got better at this each time.

I am grateful and thankful to God for sending my husband to love and to give me a wonderful family. Between us, it's just meant to be. I know how fortunate I am to have a wonderful son and the best husband in the whole wide world to cherish, love, and support me unconditionally. I have been struggling with my health problems since 1993 until now (2014). Despite all my health issues, I still have faith in God and miracles. I was baptized and became Christian in 1990, but ever since I got married, someone stopped me from continuing to practice what I believed.

I prayed for years asking God to guide me and to lead me to where I belong, and that's how I ended up at St. Gabriel the Archangel Catholic Church. I became interested in learning about the Roman Catholic Church. I attended RCIA classes at St. Gabriel the Archangel Catholic Church from September 2010 until April of 2011. At the Easter Vigil that year, I was baptized and accepted into this Catholic church and joined the communion of saints.

A few months before I converted to Catholicism, my blood pressure was elevated to over two hundred and my pulse was under fifty during the treatments at the dialysis unit. I had been monitored by the doctor and a registered nurse until I received a miracle from God at the Saturday Easter vigil. After being baptized, I didn't have these problems anymore. Amazing!

On April 15, 2011, I told my nephrologist that my goal was to reduce the blood pressure medication from six to three. He smiled at me. I was so surprised on Easter Sunday that my blood pressure was good—without taking any pills that morning. I believe it was the work of God! I got an idea about the night pills. *Maybe I don't need to take all of these pills anymore*, I thought, and therefore, I took a chance and took three pills instead of six. My goal was to come down to three blood-pressure pills each time. I hoped for the best. I kept checking my blood pressure at home—constantly—and made a list to give to my doctor as well. I was right about it! The Lord is kind and merciful.

Wow! I was impressed about what I had seen from the manual blood-pressure monitor on Monday. My blood pressure was good, and my pulse was good too. After that, both my blood pressure and my pulse were good during the treatments at the dialysis unit and at home. Now my blood pressure is under control. God is good; he is filling my heart with peace and grace. No more thinking of all the many times I felt really lonely in my heart and soul. I thank God for the miracle! I am proud to say, "I am Catholic now." I stopped questioning, *Why me?* and *Why did everything happen to me this way?*

I am proud to say that I am here to improve myself and to reform my life for life after death (eternal life). I greatly appreciate my husband for letting me do what my heart desired. Besides English, I know how to read and write Laotian and Thai.

I am very fortunate to have many good friends who cared for me through my difficult times. A tough life taught me a very expensive lesson, and I learned it the hard way—the bad feelings will follow me like a shadow, but the power of forgiveness will conquer everything, and most importantly, it gave me peace of mind. I promised myself that I would always be a good mother to my son and be a good and devoted wife to my husband forever because he is the love of my life and my destiny. Hip! Hip! Hurray! We will be celebrating our twenty-second anniversary on December 26, 2014.

Today, I still have my head up. I always have a smile on my face as if nothing much has happened to me. I have had lots of support from my mother, my family, my former teacher, my friends, especially Souvanna Kouanchao and Khonsavanh (Kay) Insisiengmay and their husbands who came to visit me while I was in the hospital. I might not be lucky with health, but I am definitely very fortunate to have these great people in my life. They will be my best friends forever.

Even with all of my friends who have helped me through my most difficult times, my greatest support has come from my husband Charlie, for being so supportive and standing by me, and the gift of my son, who has been a protector and savior in responding to critical health events that happened at home through dialing 911.

I have forgiven those people from my past who had abused me emotionally, and I have finally moved on with my life.

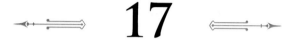

17

I love and enjoy having nephews, nieces, and the extended family members coming over to my house, especially my youngest sister. I love her, and I am very close to her. She has been very supportive through my difficult times.

During the summertime, I love to grow all kind of vegetables in my garden. I don't have to worry about the neighbors anymore! I often enjoy sharing the vegetables with my family, friends, and neighbors.

When I was younger, I fought to survive. As an adult, I fought to stay alive. The words "Fight, fight, fight" will always stay with me until the day I die.

There were two generous and wonderful ladies and one gentlemen who had stated that I was their inspiration, the first person I met at the clinic many years ago, the second and third person I met at the dialysis unit. I am privileged and honored to hear good news from them like that. I strongly believe in the virtue of faith and being a genuine and upright person. Hopefully this will take me somewhere.

I enjoy going to church two to four times per month. I have a covenant relationship with God, and I believe in one God only. I pray through Christ: "In the name of the Father, the Son, and the Holy Spirit, Amen." I volunteer at Loaves and Fishes in the city where I grew up every time I get a chance. I've enjoyed giving food to the poor and the unfortunate, something I had never done before. Then I would only hand them money. I've had a great experience and enjoyed doing volunteer work. I definitely will continue to volunteer until I can't do it any longer.

Finally, another prayer was answered. I found a reconstructive doctor for my nose. I made an appointment to see him on December 6, 2011, and I decided to have surgery on February 14, 2012. I prayed to God and kept my fingers crossed for the best result. Unfortunately, I ended up in the ICU once again after the surgery that day.

This is my destiny, and all things happened to me for a reason. It gave me the opportunity to write this story. Otherwise, I would have nothing to share or write about or even have a chance to change my life around—to be a stronger person, to have self-esteem, to be self-confident. Most importantly, it made me who I am today, and I am proud of it.

I thank God for my husband's love, honesty, and devotion. I thank God for my wonderful son. My family and I are currently living in a nice city and a good state in the US. I've repeatedly gone to dialysis on Mondays, Wednesdays, and Fridays, and dialyzed there for two and a half hours each time, so I could stay alive. I have been on a kidney-transplant list for almost nine years now, but I haven't gotten any calls. Hopefully, I'll have another chance for a kidney transplant that will last a lifetime. That will be my next journal, another chapter of my life. After recovering from the transplant, then I have to look for a job and hope for the best. My life is full of intense moments and tests of endurance, but I have no regrets.

This is a sad but amazing story about tough times and inspiration. I have written about my real life story from the bottom of my heart. Hopefully, my true life experiences will inspire the sick, both young and old, to hang tough. I want my story to be for those people who might want to give up on life to become stronger persons. To those who question if life is worth living, especially the dialysis patients, I want them to relate to my situations—to fight, to become a fighter, to be a persistent person like me.

Everything has happened to me for a reason from the above. My career goal was to become an accountant. I've never asked to have an ongoing health problems, and I never thought of becoming a writer. But I am not an accountant now. I'm having ongoing health problems, and surprisingly, I became an author of my own book by God's miracle and my destiny. Do you believe in miracles or destiny?

Oh, yes I do!